Cancer Glue for Adults

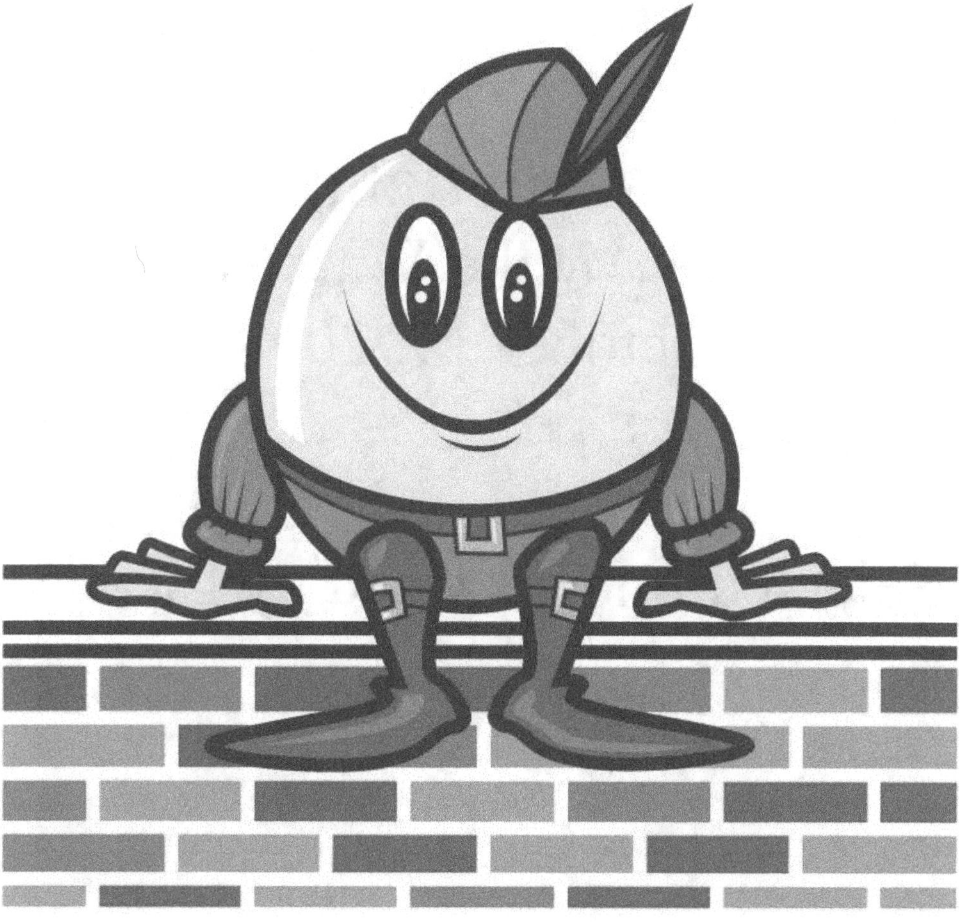

Love From Kids

Reverend Mike Wanner

Copyright
Rev. Mike Wanner
October 19, 2018

Selected Images Used by License

"Healing Presents" Tab
"Prison Presents" Tab

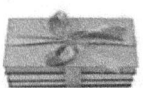

http://www.AngelRaphaelSpeaks.com

Introduction

When I was a child, my father got sick with cancer, and he had a hard time, and eventually, he was called by God, and I missed him. That was many years ago, and I wished that I could have done more for him.

I did not understand, but I wanted to, and it was impossible to know what to do to help others. I tried to comprehend but could not find answers.

The wanting to understand has influenced my life. The one thing that I remembered so firmly was the importance of kindness.

While the hospital situation back then was very complicated, I was helped tremendously by the kindness of the ambulance crews that came and soothed my father as they did the tough job of making him as comfortable as possible.

The ambulance organization that moved him was Burholme First Aid Corps Inc., and their motto was "Not For Self, But For Others."

When I came back from the United States Air Force after serving in Vietnam, I joined the volunteer organization and, now, forty plus years later I still volunteer to help others.

In 2015 I wrote a book about Burholme "Emergency Medical Kindness in the Cradle Of Liberty: Big City - Cracked Bell" as that year the Pennsylvania Dept of Health and the PEHSC named them The Best EMS Agency in Pennsylvania.

Dedication

This book is dedicated to the patients being treated for cancer, and their Healing Arts care teams including all Credentialed Caregivers of Medicine, Psychological and Psychiatric Professionals, Faith-based communities, and Complementary Care Providers.

Practitioners and Master-Teachers of the spiritual healing modalities are excellent facilitators who help to balance and soothe the active components of the emotional and mental and spiritual crises of cancer survivors. I have studied the Reiki, and the Integrated Energy Therapy® (IET) modalities extensively and am proud to associate with the practitioners and masters as often as I can.

And Family members who show up and visit who are essential as an additional level of comfort which can distract patients from their pain and struggle while bringing ideas and stories that can help bring peace of mind.

Table of Contents

Copyright 2
Introduction 3
Dedication 4
Table of Contents 5
1 - Why I am Writing This Book 6
2 - Disclaimer 7
3 - Faith Traditions Vary 8
4 - Kids Can Help Heal Adults 9
5 - Kids Can Help Heal Adults by Prayer 10
6 - Kids Can Heal by Smiling 12
7 - Kids Can Heal by Loving 13
8 - Kids May Help With Hands-On Healing 15
9 - Kids Can Heal by Sharing 17
10 - Kids Can Heal by Story Telling 18
11 - Kids Can Help Healing by Little Tasks 19
12 - Kids Can Help Healing by Being Quiet 20
13 - Kid Can Help Healing By Asking Good Questions 21
14 - Don't Worry Ever Kids 22
15 - Thank You 23
16 - Cancer Books by Rev. Mike 24
17 - Books Category Resources 25
18 - Angels Please Prayers 26
19 - Private Channeling 27
20 - Reverend Mike Wanner 28

1 - Why I am Writing This Book

You can read above that I have moved towards support in as many ways as I can. I write a lot about healing, and my ministry of healing messages continues to come full circle.

I just received the Our Journey of Hope training at Cancer Treatment Center of Philadelphia and learned some more about what is possible to help those in the struggle of cancer.

With this book, I would like to share with the children of today those things that I did not know so they can help soothe the adults in their life that are struggling now as my father did then. It is my hope that the time that your loved one might have left be as wonderful as possible so that both you and they embrace the gift from God that you are to each other.

Love expressed in the love from God is Blessed by your words so that the beauty and healing within the words leave Divine energy in the lives of you both.

2 - Disclaimer

I, the author, am not involved with clinical cancer care but I have talked to many cancer patients during decades of pre-hospital ambulance care and transportation and also many years of Hospital Pastoral Care. I am sharing what is coming to me in an effort to spread understanding and trigger conversation that can be helpful. It may be that the discussion needs finessing and I invite your wisdom into the mix.

My guidance has suggested that a lot can be done to soothe the times for cancer patients and their families. I will detail my views which are not the expert positions of a Cancer Center Clinician or technician or social worker, or Medical Practitioner or Psychologist or Psychiatrist or another expert who might be helpful here.

I have said, everything about cancer may seem very complicated, but there are always simple and practical ideas that can be embraced when a person is open to see common sense items that are within their capability. Please be diligent and check with attending nurses and physicians before doing anything that might in any way violate care protocols. If in doubt, ask enough to know.

Please also be diligent about what you share with the patient so that they are not stressed by overwhelming information that they cannot process. The ideal medicine or process that helped someone in your world may not be appropriate for the person you are talking with, so please leave medicine to the Doctor and the technicians.

3 - Faith Traditions Vary

Adults are invited to please be aware that faith traditions vary and some words here written may not be perfectly aligned with the beliefs of a child's parents. Parents reading this in advance of sharing is recommended to avoid any confusion.

If you are concerned about interpretations, please advise so that I can consider your suggestions to simplify the messages.

Please be aware of the age and feelings of all listeners.

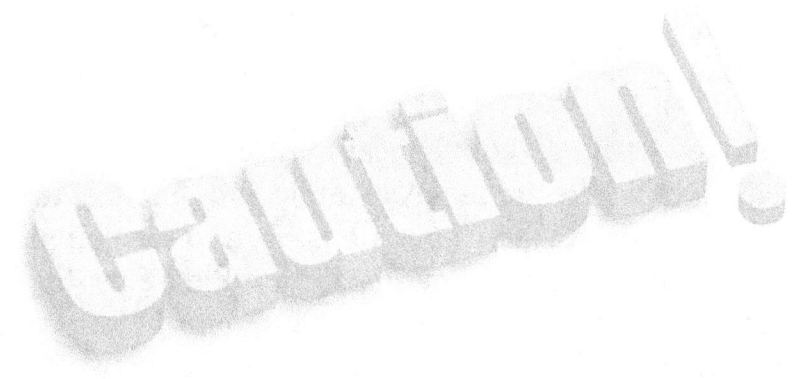

4 - Kids Can Help Heal Adults

Children can do many things to help adults heal, and they can do it without a lot of work.

Children can help adults heal with:

>Prayer
>
>Smiles
>
>Loving
>
>Hands-On Healing
>
>Sharing
>
>Telling Stories
>
>Doing Little Tasks
>
>Being Quiet when asked
>
>Asking Good Questions

5 - Kids Can Help Heal Adults by Prayer

A simple way to pray is to Recognize God, Unify with God, Claim to heal as if it is already started, Acknowledge the healing, and Thank God for the Healing. When we pray, we request the beginning of healing which can grow as we continue to pray every day. When we say "Thy Will Be Done," We accept God's view of what is right.

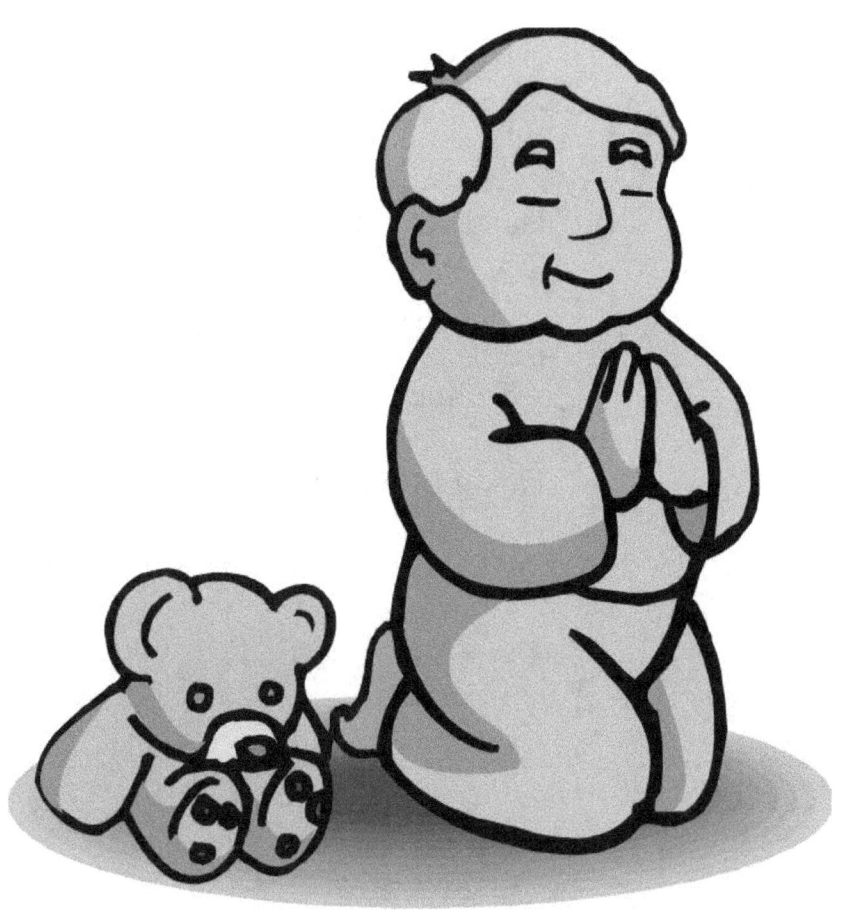

Hello God

Hello God this is _____

I want to pray for _____

Prayer Example

I/ we recognize you as the Source of All Good, All Healing, Everything, and Everyone.

I/we claim my/our unification with you Now!

I/we claim healing for any appearance of
(what)_____ in
(who)_____, Now.

I/we acknowledge the healing is already in process, Now

I/we thank you God for this healing and all our blessings as we say – AND SO IT IS! Amen and Amen.

6 - Kids Can Heal by Smiling

Try not to be stingy with your smiles.

When someone is sick, they may not smile
And
that can make you sad.

When you are sad, that may make them sadder
And
That does not help them heal.

Sad is not good for healing.

If you are sad and visit someone sick;

1. Please Pray First

2. Please Smile Second

7 - Kids Can Heal by Loving

Try not to be stingy with your Love.

When someone is sick, they may not feel loved
And
that can make you sad.

When you are sad, you may want them to feel loved
And
You Can Say I Love You.

When they feel your love, sad can go away.

If you are sad and visit someone sick:

Please Pray

Please Smile

Please Say I Love You

8 - Kids May Help With Hands-On Healing

Jesus declared that the work that he does, you can also do if you believe in him.

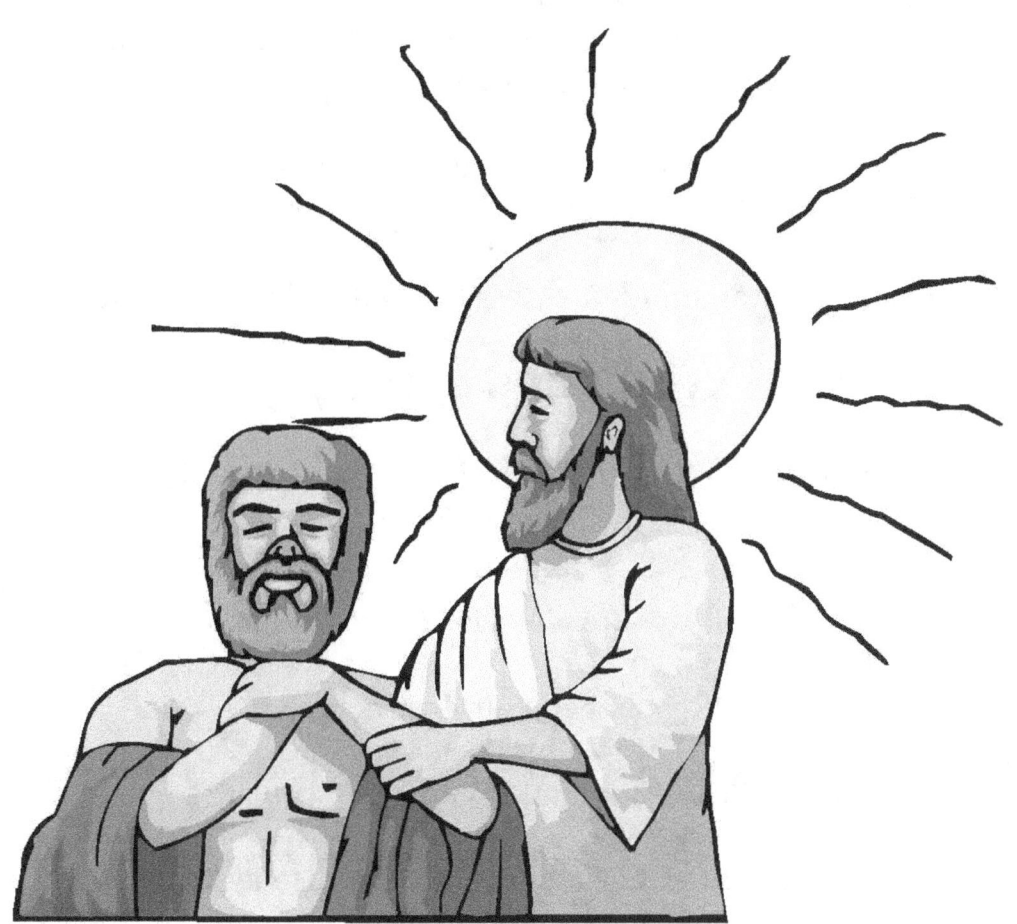

Children can lay their hands on the sick if they are careful and get permission from the one they love who is ill and also the Doctors or the Nurses.

John 14.10 '…I speak not of myself: but the father that dwelleth in me, he doeth the works. "

John 14.12 "…I say unto you, He that believeth on me, the works that I do shall he do also: and greater works than these shall he do; because I go unto my father."

John 14.18 "I will not leave you comfortless: I will come to you."

*

Mark 9:23 " …all things are possible to him that believeth."

Start With A Prayer

Dear God, Please Bless This Special One Now
(Example Above)

Make Sure You Have Permission

Remember Your Instructions

Please Be Gentle With Your Touch

Please Be Careful With Your Hands

Smile As You Pray

9 - Kids Can Heal by Sharing

Sharing with your friends can help you, and the loved one you have been praying for because your friends can pray for you and your loved one. It also allows people to feel they belong when someone shares a secret with them even if it makes them a little sad for a little while.

Friends can help to understand you and help you feel that you are supported and befriended. Deep down many people want to help others, but they do not want to intrude in your life.

When you share, you open yourself to a larger community of opportunities and support,

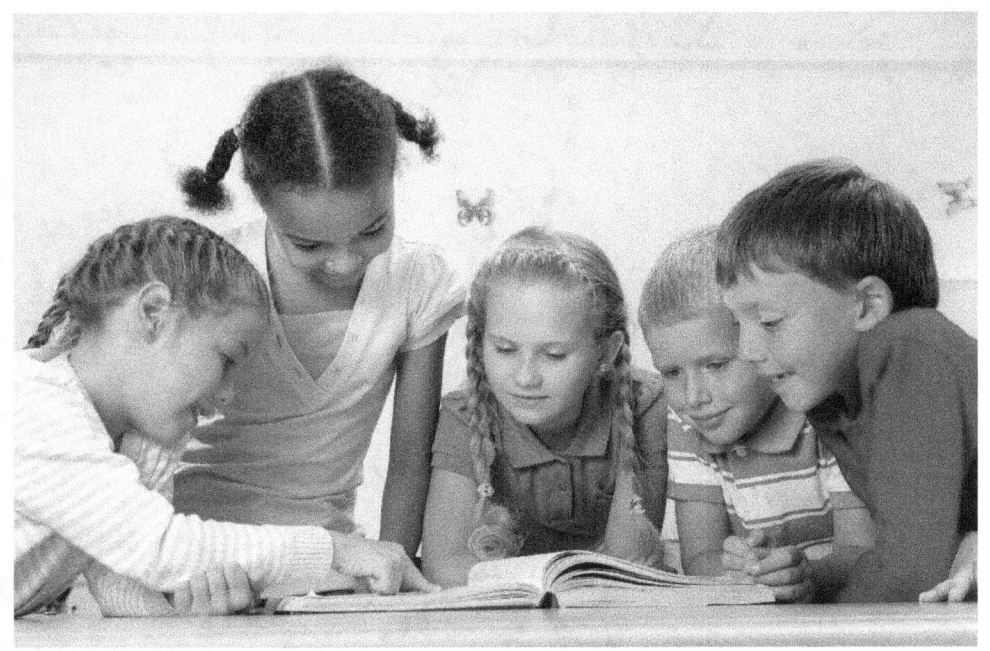

10 - Kids Can Heal by Story Telling

When people are interested in you, they ask questions. Sometimes that may not feel so good, and we may want to cheer them up so we can tell a story to them.

The story can be from a book, or it can be the story of your week, your month or your year. It can also be the story of the plan for your life.

You can talk about anything or anyone that might be interested in learning about. You invite them into your world.

When you bring them into your world, you disrupt the reality that is not serving them well.

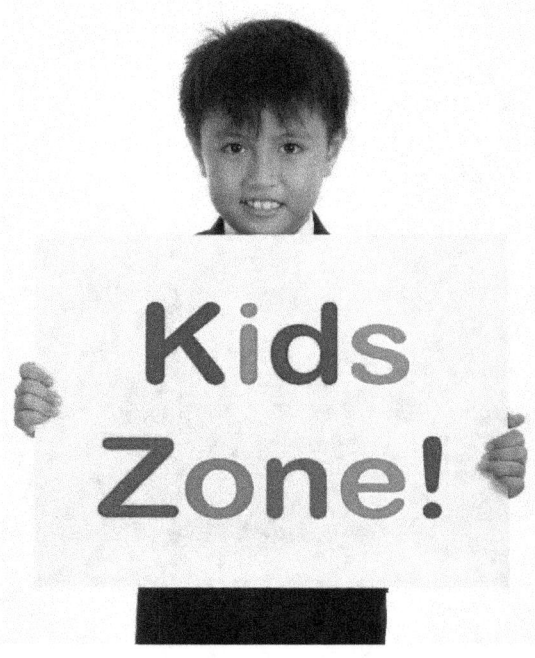

11 - Kids Can Help Healing by Little Tasks

Family members who are sick may not want to trouble you for help with little things. When they do not ask, you do not know.

You can make it a habit of asking what you can do to help. Little things can help a lot, consider asking about things:

1. Do You need your Medicine?

2. Do You need the telephone?

3. Do You need your sweater?

4. Can I Help with anything?

5. Would you like some water?

6. Would you like a tissue.?

7. Would you like me to call the nurse?

8. Would you like me to cut your food?

12 - Kids Can Help Healing by Being Quiet

When too many things are happening at the same time, adults can become upset without reason. They may ask you to be quiet, and if you can , it would be fantastic.

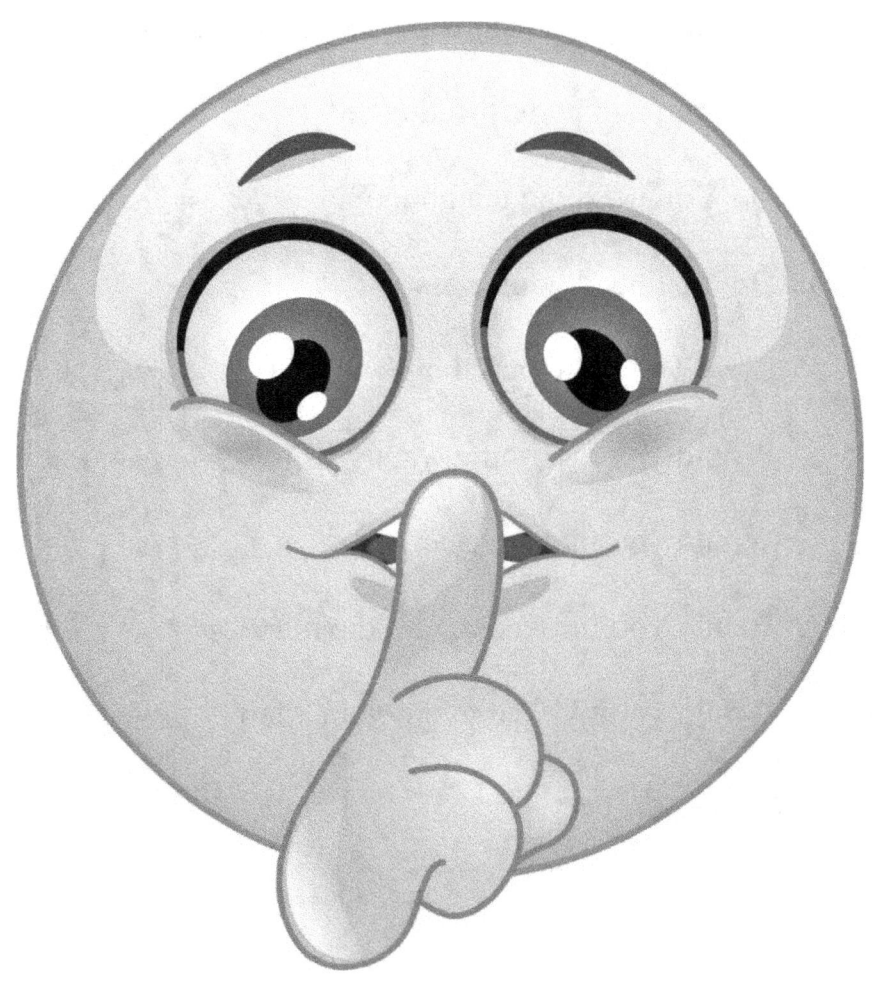

13 - Kid Can Help Healing By Asking Good Questions

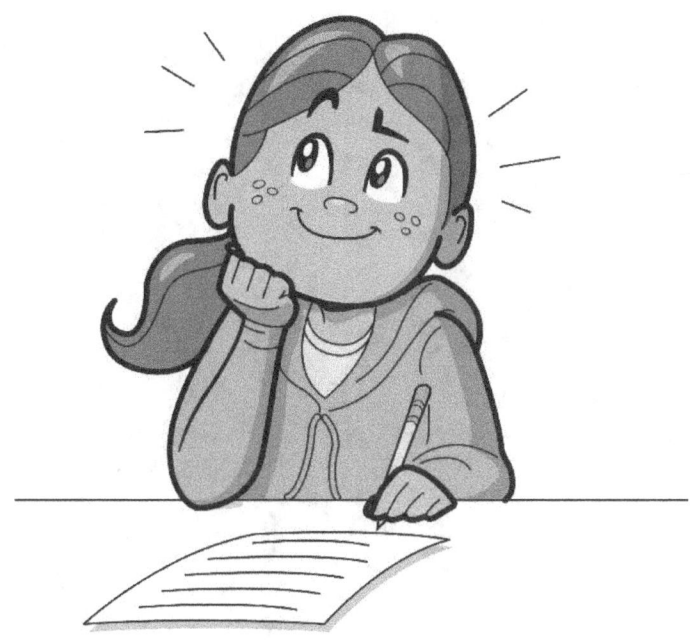

Think About your Question

Write it Down

Ask an Adult who is not sick if your question is gentle

If the answer is Yes, You can Ask.

14 - Don't Worry Ever Kids

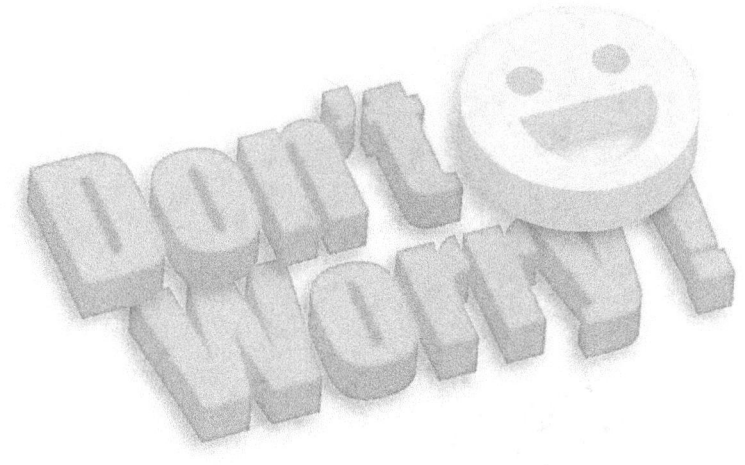

Ever

It Does Not Help Prayer Still Does!

Resource: http://Create-A-Prayer.com

15 - Thank You

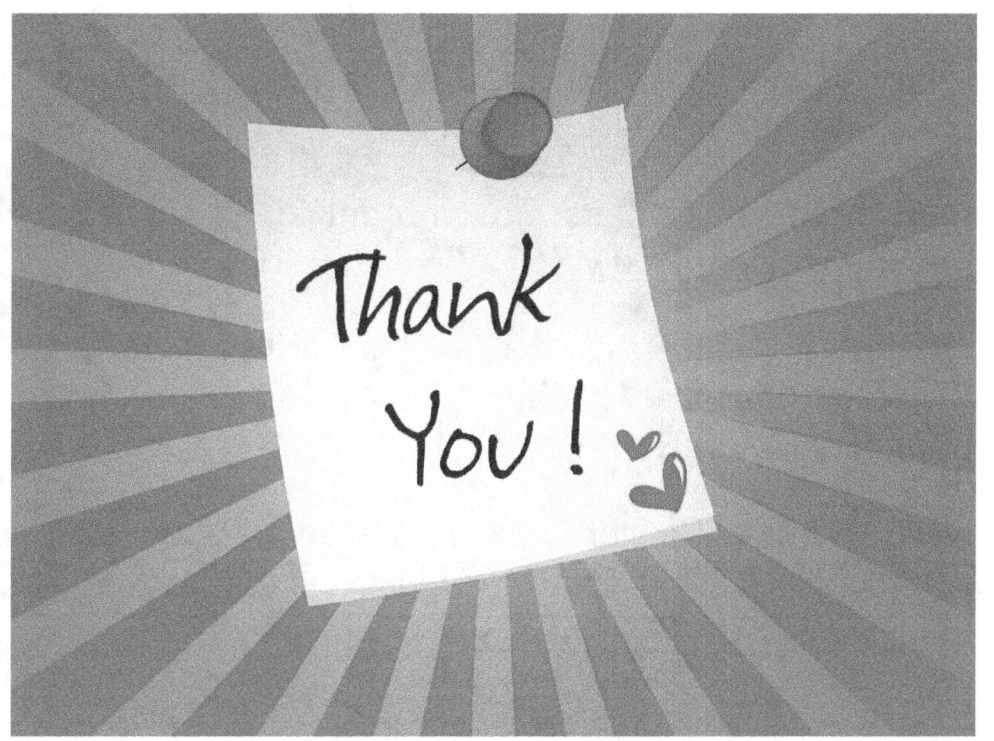

For
Considering
These
Ideas

16 - Cancer Books by Rev. Mike

Cancer Glue For Adults: Love From Reiki
http://amzn.com/B07JQPBWW6

Cancer Glue For Adults: Love From Kids
http://amzn.com/B00MS6M77I

Does Reiki Love Heal Cancer?: Transcribed True Stories Of Spiritual Healing
http://amzn.com/B00MS6M77I

Reiki Help For Cancer Care in Pottstown, PA: Cecilia Appreciates PMMC Cancer Center
http://amzn.com/B071XBTSFX

Reiki For Cancer
http://amzn.com/B07873YKLJ

17 - Books Category Resources at www.Amazon.com

Distant Healing (or Mail List) e-mail mikewann@voicenet.com

Veterans Healing Six Pack plus 2
http://angelraphaelspeaks.com/healing-books/veterans/

PTSD Power Pack
http://angelraphaelspeaks.com/healing-books/ptsd/

Angel Raphael Speaks Series & Other Angel Books
http://angelraphaelspeaks.com/

Reiki
http://angelraphaelspeaks.com/healing-books/reiki/

Children
http://angelraphaelspeaks.com/healing-books/children/

Emergency Medical Kindness
http://angelraphaelspeaks.com/healing-books/emergency-medical-kindness/

Cancer
http://angelraphaelspeaks.com/healing-books/cancer/

Addictions
http://angelraphaelspeaks.com/healing-books/addictions/

Miscellaneous Healing
http://angelraphaelspeaks.com/healing-books/misc-healing/

Prison Books - 50+ Prison Books
http://angelraphaelspeaks.com/prison-books/

18 - Angels Please Prayers

Addict's
Angels of Healing Selected
Help Me to Stay Directed
Come To Me From The Sky
I Am Ready to Succeed Not Try
If I Don't Invite You In
I Might Not Win
I Have Been Lost For Too Long
Help Me To Stay Strong

Alcoholic's
Angels of Healing On High
Help Me to Stay Dry
Come To Me From The Sky
I Am Ready to Succeed Not Try
If I Don't Invite You In
I Might Not Win
I Have Been Lost For Too Long
Help Me To Stay Strong

Prayers Above From

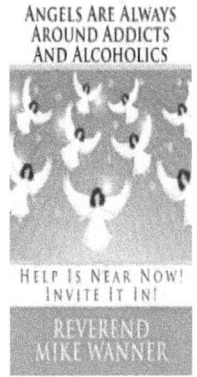

http://AngelRaphaelSpeaks.com/AAAAAA/
The Link Above Has the Core Messages from the book on drop-down pages.

19 - Private Channeling

Angel Raphael Speaks a series of free messages that are channeled through Reverend Mike Wanner for the Highest good and Highest Healing of all concerned.

Many questions arise about Reverend Mike doing private channeling, and he does help with that so E-mail him.

Reverend Mike is available worldwide as a psychic channel, emotional release facilitator, spiritual energy practitioner & teacher, and public speaker.

He looks forward to meeting you soon! Email - mikewann@voicenet.com 215-342-1270

PRIVATE SPIRITUAL READINGS/channelings or Spiritual Healing Sessions: Telephone or in person.

Rev. Mike is available for individual, intuitive one-on-one sessions with you, his Guide Family, and your Guides. He helps by offering clarity on emotional situations about your life, your purpose, your spirituality, and your release of stuffed emotions and cellular memory.

Connect to the love of your Guides today!

For more information, Please visit

http://angelraphaelspeaks.com/channel/

20 - Reverend Mike Wanner

Rev. Mike Wanner started his spiritual and ministerial studies with Reiki in 1993 and had studied seven styles of Reiki in the U.S., Japan, Canada, Denmark, and Australia. He is certified to teach.

He became certified to teach Integrated Energy Therapy in 1999 and co-taught the first IET class of the new Millennium. Mike began dowsing in 2001.

Ordained as an Interfaith Minister of the Circle of Miracles Ministry and a Metaphysical Minister of the International Metaphysical Ministry, Rev. Mike practices and teaches spiritual energy therapies in the Philadelphia Area.

Rev. Mike holds ministerial degrees from the University of Metaphysics and the University of Sedona. He is a Pastoral Care Associate at Jefferson - Frankford Hospital. He taught at the National Academy of Massage Therapy and Health Sciences.

Rev. Mike was a faculty member of the Medical Mission Sister's Center for Human Integration's School of Integrated Body/Mind Therapies in Fox Chase, Philadelphia, PA for twelve years.

For a complete Biography, Please visit

http://ReverendMikeWanner.com/Bio